Stay Safe From Cancer: Expert Tips And Advice For Prevention

Looking for ways to help lower your cancer risk and improve your overall health? Learn more about proven modifiable risk factors

By

Solomon Jefferson

All Right Reserved

TABLE OF CONTENTS

Presentation

Cancer continues to be a global health crisis, with the number of cases on a steady rise worldwide. Because of its startling increase in occurrence, cancer has become the most pressing public health concern. Whether through personal experiences or the shocking statistics that dominate headlines, it is impossible to ignore the impact that cancer has on people and societies.

Imagine this: Cancer kills millions of people annually, destroying families and changing lives in the process. The reality is all too grim, with one in three people being diagnosed with cancer at some point in their lives. According to the World Health Organisation (WHO), cancer is responsible for almost one in six deaths globally. It is among the leading causes of death in the world.

The statistics have reached a staggering rate. Approximately 700,000 people die from cancer in Africa each year, out of 1.1 million new cases. If immediate action is not taken, data estimates indicate that the annual death toll from cancer will rise significantly to about one million by 2030.

The need and urgency of cancer prevention are aptly illustrated by these statistics. In short, this fact serves as a sobering reminder that everyone is vulnerable to it and that early detection is important. Now is the time for us to take charge of our health and prevent this terrible disease by arming ourselves with expert tips and advice that help us stay safe from this devastating disease.

This book is more than just another book on cancer. It is a comprehensive guide that combines scientific research, expert opinions, and practical advice to educate people. It is a call to action, an invitation to join the fight against cancer by taking charge of our own lives.

In the chapters that follow, we will explore the complexities of cancer, looking at how it develops and the reasons behind various types, including skin, colon, lung, breast, and prostate cancer. By exploring the prevalence rates and statistics associated with these cancers, we hope to paint a comprehensive picture of the magnitude of this global health crisis.

In each chapter, we will cover topics such as assessing vulnerability to cancer, the impact of environmental and work-related factors, the dangers of alcohol and tobacco use, and the need to engage in regular physical exercise. We will discuss protective measures, practical steps, and prevention strategies tailored to specific types of cancer.

Cancer is a public health issue of major concern. We cannot underestimate the power of knowledge and prevention when it comes to protecting ourselves from cancer. This work gives you an all-inclusive guide that will enable you to take control of your health and maintain a cancer-free lifestyle through professional advice and extensive research. It calls for the unification of like-minded people as we build new and innovative alliances and collaborative efforts in the fight against cancer. Together, let us work towards a healthier, safer future.

Foreword

Cancer is a deadly disease that knows no boundaries and kills people at an alarming rate all around the world. Globally, the cancer epidemic is still getting worse, putting a great deal of physical, psychological, and financial hardship on people, families, communities, and health systems. Many low- and middle-income countries lack the necessary health systems to handle this problem, and many cancer patients worldwide lack access to timely, high-quality diagnosis and treatment. In countries with advanced health systems, survival rates of different types of cancers are improving — thanks to their sophisticated health systems.

As the number of cases increases, we must empower ourselves with knowledge and precautions to stay ahead of the curve. The first line of defence against cancer is prevention, and with this book, we intend to provide comprehensive guidelines and ways to help lower your cancer risk and improve your overall health based on in-depth research and analysis.

Every day, we are confronted with startling statistics and heart-wrenching personal stories that shed light on the devastating impact of cancer. According to recent studies, cancer claims millions of lives each year and is currently one of the leading causes of mortality worldwide. The need to adopt proactive measures beforehand cannot be overstated, as this fact serves as a sobering reminder that everyone is at risk of it.

Of course! This is a personal story that emphasises the importance of cancer prevention: A close friend of mine lost her brother to lung cancer a few years ago. Her brother had been a heavy smoker for most of his life, and despite the numerous warnings and known risks associated with smoking, he was unable to quit. By the time his lung cancer was diagnosed, it had already reached an advanced stage and spread to other organs, making treatment options limited. This terrible incident made clear how important it is to prevent cancer, especially when it comes to giving up risk factors like smoking, which can significantly increase one's chance of developing cancer.

According to statistics from the World Health Organisation (WHO), approximately one-third of cancer cases that are diagnosed each year can be attributed to preventable causes. This shocking statistic emphasises how important cancer preventive strategies are and how much of an impact they may have in reducing the global burden of cancer. Implementing and promoting lifestyle changes like quitting smoking, maintaining a healthy diet, and practising safe behaviour around known carcinogens, and environmental and occupational hazards can help prevent many cancer cases and save countless lives.

With the information in this work, we can take control of our health, adopt preventive measures and reduce our risk of this devastating disease. Several factors make this book unique in its comprehensive approach to providing expert tips and advice for cancer prevention: The book is written by renowned doctors, researchers, and experts in the field of oncology. They provide their extensive knowledge and expertise to offer evidence-based guidance on cancer prevention. The book incorporates the latest scientific research on cancer prevention. To ensure that the advice and recommendations are backed up by facts, it compiles information from reputable sources and medical journals.

The book provides thorough explanations of every element—genetics, lifestyle choices, environmental variables, and more — that affects the development of cancer. This comprehensive approach enables readers to have a clear understanding of cancer prevention. This book not only provides information but also offers practical tips and recommendations that people can incorporate into their daily lives. It provides advice on how to modify one's food, engage in physical activity, alter one's lifestyle, and use other tried-and-true cancer prevention methods.

Finally, this book aims to create awareness of the various types of cancer and the risk factors associated with them. It provides readers with the information they need to actively prevent cancer by stressing the need for self-examinations, routine screenings, and early detection.

Chapter 1

Explanation of what cancer is and how it develops

Cancer, a word that strikes fear into the hearts of many, is a disease in which some of the body's cells grow uncontrollably and spread to other parts of the body. These abnormal cells, commonly known as cancer cells, can impair the regular operation of the tissues and organs around them. If cancer is not identified and treated on time, it may metastasize, or spread to other parts of the body. This would complicate the course of treatment.

Before cancer appears, one cell may experience several genetic changes. These changes can be caused by a variety of factors, such as viral infections, exposure to particular environmental toxins or chemicals, and inherited gene mutations. Because of these genetic changes, the cell may eventually become incapable of regulating its division and development. The cell consequently starts to divide and expand swiftly, eventually turning into a tumour.

There are two main types of tumours: benign and malignant. Benign tumours are not cancerous and frequently stay inside of their original location. Benign tumours do not penetrate or spread to other tissues in the vicinity. Benign tumours often don't grow back after removal, while cancerous tumours can. But benign tumours can grow to be rather enormous at times. Some, like benign brain tumours, are potentially fatal or cause severe symptoms.

However, malignant tumours are cancerous and can spread to other parts of the body through the lymphatic or circulatory systems, infecting nearby tissues. This process, known as metastasis, is a major factor in why cancer is so difficult to treat.

Discussion of different types of cancers and their causes

Lung Cancer

Lung cancer is a type of cancer that starts when abnormal cells grow in an uncontrolled way in the lungs. It is a serious health problem that can cause severe harm and death. The two main organs that make up the lungs are located beneath the rib cage and above the diaphragm. Your lungs take up oxygen while breathing and transfer it to the bloodstream, which then distributes it throughout the body. The lungs eliminate carbon dioxide, a waste gas, from the bloodstream when you breathe out. Breathing becomes more challenging when lung cancer obstructs this essential function.

Lung cancer is one of the deadliest cancers and is primarily caused by long-term tobacco use, especially secondhand smoke. Exposure to radon gas, asbestos, or particular industrial chemicals could be an additional risk factor

Lung cancer can cause several symptoms that may indicate a problem in the lungs. The most common symptoms include:
cough that does not go away
chest pain
shortness of breath
lung infections that keep coming back.
fatigue
coughing up blood (haemoptysis)
weight loss with no known cause

Early symptoms may be mild or dismissed as common respiratory issues, leading to delayed diagnosis.

Breast Cancer
Breast cancer is more common in women, but it can also affect men. Breast cancer is a condition where abnormal breast cells proliferate and develop into tumours. Tumours can become dangerous if they

proliferate throughout the body and are not treated. Inside the breast's milk ducts and/or milk-producing lobules are where breast cancer cells first proliferate. It is not difficult to deal with during the early stage. But if left untreated cancer cells can invade nearby breast tissue. This creates tumours that cause lumps or thickening.

About 80% of breast cancer cases are invasive, meaning a tumour may spread from your breast to other areas of your body. While women over 50 are more likely to get breast cancer than men, younger women can also develop breast cancer. Breast cancer may affect men and women equally. Healthcare providers may treat breast cancer with surgery to remove tumours or treatment to kill cancerous cells.

Causes of Breast Cancer
Experts understand that breast cancer develops from a mutation in breast cells that turns them into cancerous cells that

proliferate and divide to form tumours. They are not sure of what causes that change. However, studies indicate that some factors could raise your risk of breast cancer. Among these are:

A family history of the disease
Drinking beverages containing alcohol
Inherited genetic mutations
Age — being 55 or older
Smoking
Radiation exposure
Hormone replacement therapy.

What Are the Symptoms of Breast Cancer?

Breast cancer can have different symptoms for different people. Some people don't notice any signs at all. Common symptoms of breast cancer include:

A lump in your breast or underarm that doesn't go away is one of the common signs of breast cancer. Frequently, this is the initial sign of breast cancer. Typically, a lump on a breast can be detected by your doctor much before you can.

Swelling in your armpit or near your collarbone. This may indicate that the breast cancer has progressed to the nearby lymph nodes. Inform your doctor of any swelling you observe, as it may begin before you feel a bump.

A change in the appearance of your skin on your breast or nipple. Your skin may look dimpled, puckered, scaly or inflamed. It may look red, purple or darker than other parts of your breast.

Breast changes such as a difference in the size, contour, texture, or temperature of your breast.

Changes to your nipple, such as one that:
Draws inward
Has a dimple

Burns and Itches

Grows sores

Unusual discharge from the nipples.

Breast Cancer in Men

Men have some breast tissue even though their breasts are smaller than women's. The breasts of a girl before puberty are comparable to the "breasts" of a male. Men's tissue does not grow and develop like that of girls'.

However, men are susceptible to breast cancer because they still have breast tissue. The same forms of breast cancers that affect women also affect men, however, those that affect the organs that produce and retain milk are uncommon. The risk of a man getting breast cancer in his lifetime is about 1 per 1,000.

The main problem is that male breast cancer is frequently detected later than female breast cancer. This might be the case because men are less inclined to suspect something strange in that area.

Symptoms of Male Breast cancer
Men develop breast cancer at a rate of about 1%. You might not notice the signs until the cancer has spread because it is not a common problem. Watch out for:

A thick spot or lump under your armpit or breast.
changes to your breast or nipple skin, like redness, puckering, scaling, or discharge.

Prostate Cancer
Prostate cancer is the cancer that affects the prostate. In men, the prostate is a tiny, walnut-shaped gland that secretes the seminal fluid that carries and nourishes sperm.

Prostate cancer is among the most prevalent cancers. Many prostate cancers develop in the prostate gland, where they may not spread quickly and may not be very harmful. But while some forms of prostate cancer spread quickly, others develop slowly and may require little to no treatment at all.

The probability of a successful outcome for prostate cancer treatment is early detection, while the cancer is still limited to the prostate gland. Prostate cancer is more commonly diagnosed in older men. Risk factors include age, family history, weight, race (African Americans have a higher risk of this kind of cancer), and particular genetic abnormalities.

Prostate cancer may cause no signs or symptoms in its early stages. A prostate cancer that has developed may cause signs and symptoms such as:

Trouble urinating

Decreased force in the stream of urine
Blood in the urine
Blood in the semen
Bone pain
Losing weight without trying
Erectile dysfunction

When to see a doctor?
Make an appointment with your doctor if you have any persistent signs or symptoms that worry you.

Colorectal cancer

Colorectal cancer also called Colon cancer is the growth of cells that begins in a part of the large intestine called the colon. The colon is the first and longest part of the large intestine. Colon cancer may affect anyone at any age, but it usually affects older people. Usually, it starts as little groups of cells inside the colon called polyps. Polyps generally aren't cancerous, but some can turn into colon cancers over time.

Polyps frequently show no symptoms. Doctors advise routine screening tests to check for colon polyps because of this. Finding and removing polyps helps prevent colon cancer.

If colon cancer develops, many therapies can help in dealing with it. Among the treatments include radiation therapy, surgery, and medications like immunotherapy, chemotherapy, and targeted therapy.

Colorectal cancer is another name for colon cancer. This phrase refers to cancer that starts in the rectum and includes both colon and rectal cancer.

Colorectal cancer might not cause symptoms right away, but if it does, it may cause one or more of these symptoms:
A change in bowel habits, such as more frequent diarrhoea or constipation.
Rectal bleeding or blood in the stool.

Ongoing discomfort in the belly area, such as cramps, gas or pain.
A feeling that the bowel doesn't empty during a bowel movement.
Weakness or tiredness.
Losing weight without trying.

Age, family history, inflammatory bowel disease, certain genetic abnormalities, a diet high in red or processed meats, low intake of fibre, smoking, diabetes, obesity, inflammatory bowel diseases and excessive alcohol use are just a few of the many factors that may be involved in the development of colorectal cancer, which affects the colon or rectum.

Skin cancer and melanoma
Skin cancer usually appears on sun-exposed parts of the skin, such as the scalp, face, lips, ears, neck, chest, arms, and hands. It can also develop in the areas of your body that are never exposed to daylight.

People with darker skin tones are not immune to the effects of skin cancer. Dark-skinned people are more likely to develop melanoma on parts of their bodies like the palms of their hands and the soles of their feet that are shielded from the sun.

By reducing or eliminating your exposure to ultraviolet (UV) radiation, you can lower your risk of developing skin cancer. Early detection of skin cancer can be achieved by continually watching your skin for any unusual changes. Early detection of skin cancer gives you the greatest chance for successful skin cancer treatment.

Signs and symptoms of skin cancer
In its early stages, skin cancer frequently shows no symptoms, however, it might develop at any time. A change on your skin, either a new growth or a modification to an existing growth or mole, is the most prevalent warning sign of skin cancer. The following are symptoms of skin cancer:

A new spot on the skin or changes in the size, shape or colour of an existing spot. These changes can vary greatly so there is no one way to describe how a skin cancer looks.

A spot that is itchy or painful

A non-healing sore that bleeds or develops a crust

A red rough or scaly spot that you can feel

A growth with a raised border and central crust or bleeding

A wart-like growth

A wound or sore that won't heal, or that heals but comes back again.

A scar-like growth without a well-defined border

If you're worried about a mole or another skin lesion, consult your doctor. They'll examine your skin and may ask you to see a dermatologist and have the lesion further evaluated.

What are the risk factors for skin cancer?

Although anyone can develop skin cancer, your chances are high if you:

Have been exposed to UV light therapy for treating skin conditions such as eczema or psoriasis.

Have many moles or irregularly shaped moles.

Take medications that suppress or weaken your immune system.

Spend a considerable amount of time working or playing in the sun.

Have a family history of skin cancer.

Get easily sunburned or have a history of sunburns.

Live in a sunny or high-altitude climate.

Tan or use tanning beds.

Have had an organ transplant.

Other common types of cancer

There are numerous other types of cancer, each with specific causes and risk factors. These include leukaemia as well as cancers of the bladder, kidney, ovary, cervix, and pancreas, among others.

Statistics and prevalence rates

Cancers are one of the leading causes of death globally. Cancer is one of the world's largest health problems. Almost 10 Million people die from cancer annually. The Global Burden of Disease estimates that every sixth death in the world is due to cancer, making it the second leading cause of death – second only to cardiovascular diseases. Because cancer is one of the leading causes of death, it is one of the world's most pressing problems to make progress against this disease.

Female breast cancer has surpassed lung cancer as the most commonly diagnosed cancer, followed by lung, colorectal, prostate, and stomach cancers. Lung cancer remained the leading cause of cancer death, followed by colorectal, liver, stomach, and female breast cancers. It is critical to keep in mind that survival rates vary greatly depending on the stage of cancer diagnosis, highlighting the need for early detection and preventive actions.

This is a very personal topic to many: nearly everyone knows or has lost someone dear to them from this disease. Based on factors like age, gender, location, and lifestyle, the prevalence of some cancers varies. As the share of people with cancer increases globally people and communities should see the need to make progress against cancer and many other causes of deaths

This chapter looks at the causes of different types of cancer, the complexity of how cancer develops, and the startling statistics and prevalence rates. It establishes the foundation for the remaining chapters in the book. With this knowledge in hand, we can work to prevent cancer and move closer to the day when it won't be a worldwide health crisis.

Chapter 2

Early Detection and Screening

Screening can often help find and treat pre-cancers and cancers early before they have a chance to spread. Finding cancer early and getting treatment are two of the most important strategies for preventing deaths from cancer. Cancer that's found at its early stage when it has not spread, will be easy to treat. Getting regular screening tests is the most reliable way to find cancer early. This chapter provides details on the importance of early detection and screening test recommendations by age.

Importance of Early Detection

Cancer that's diagnosed at an early stage, when it isn't too large and hasn't spread, is more likely to be treated successfully. Many types of cancer are now completely treatable, even though most people find the thought of having cancer to be scary. Notably, there are a lot of people who have survived cancer, particularly in developed nations like the US and Europe. Studies have shown that advancements in technology, detection and diagnostic tools, and genetic testing have all contributed to a decrease in the death rate among cancer patients. These advancements have increased the possibility of an effective treatment by improving the early detection of abnormal cells before they develop into cancerous ones.

Diagnosing cancer when it hasn't spread means that treatment is more likely to be successful. Reducing diseases and cancer-related deaths is the goal of screening. People who are at risk or concerned about cancer can benefit from this approach. This is important as it is one of the first actions taken to prevent the disease. It is crucial to notify your doctor right away if you see anything that isn't typical for you because early detection saves lives.

Early diagnosis of breast cancer

Breast cancers discovered by screening are more likely to be small and to have not spread outside of the breast. One of the most important factors in determining a woman's prognosis for breast cancer is the size of the tumour and the extent of its dissemination.

These guidelines are for women whose risk of breast cancer is average. For screening purposes, a woman is deemed to be at average risk if she has not had chest radiation therapy before the age of 30, has no personal history of breast cancer, has a strong family history of breast cancer, or has a genetic mutation known to increase risk of breast cancer (such as in a BRCA gene).

Screening recommendations for women at average breast cancer risk

- Women between the ages of 40 and 44 should be able to begin yearly screenings for breast cancer using mammograms, or x-rays of the breast.

- Women between the ages of 45 and 54 ought to have annual mammograms.

- Women 55 and older should switch to mammograms every 2 years or can continue yearly screening.

- As long as a woman is in excellent health and is anticipated to survive for at least another ten years, screening should continue.

- The benefits, limitations, and possible risks associated with breast cancer screening should be known by all women.

- Additionally, women should be aware of the typical appearance and shape of their breasts and promptly report any changes to a healthcare professional.

Some women should get MRIs in addition to mammograms as part of their screening process due to family history, genetic predisposition, or other reasons. (There are relatively few women that fit this description.) Discuss your risk for breast cancer and the most appropriate screening plan with a medical professional.

Globally, women are diagnosed with breast cancer more often than any other cancer. Mammography screening is the gold standard for early breast cancer identification when the disease is most treatable. Mammograms should normally be obtained every one to two years by women between the ages of 40 and 74. In addition to self-examinations, medical experts can undertake clinical breast examinations to detect breast abnormalities.

Prostate Cancer Screening Guidelines
Because it grows slowly and remains inside the prostate gland, prostate cancer frequently has no symptoms. However, treatment is required for some forms of prostate cancer that spread swiftly. By detecting the disease early on, when it is

easier to treat routine screening can reduce your chance of dying from prostate cancer.

Cancer that grows slowly can potentially be detected by screening. Some people may be alarmed by this type of cancer and may end up receiving unnecessary therapy. Other people might feel at ease treating this low-risk prostate cancer without getting medical attention.

What is the screening test for prostate cancer?
Screening for prostate cancer is done with a simple blood test called a prostate-specific antigen (PSA) test. This test quantifies the amount of protein in your blood that is by prostate gland cells. If you have a prostate issue, your PSA levels will increase. It's normal to have a low level of PSA.

What is the Screening Protocol for Prostate Cancer Early Detection

The American Cancer Society recommends that men make an informed decision with a healthcare provider about whether to be tested for prostate cancer.

- Starting at age 50, men should talk to a healthcare provider about the pros and cons of testing so they can decide if testing is the right choice for them.

- If you are African American or have a father or brother who had prostate cancer before age 65, you should have this talk with a healthcare provider starting at age 45.

- If you decide to be tested, you should get a PSA blood test with or without a rectal exam. How often you're tested will depend on your PSA level

The choices you make about what you eat, how active you are, and other behaviours can affect your overall health as well as your chance of developing cancer and other serious diseases.

Screening guidelines for colorectal cancer?

The American Cancer Society suggests beginning routine screening for colorectal cancer at age 45 for those who are at average risk of the disease. This can be done either with a sensitive test that looks for signs of cancer in a person's stool (a stool-based test) or with an exam that looks at the colon and rectum (a visual exam). Getting tested is the most essential thing, regardless of the test you select.

- If you're in good health, you should continue regular screening through age 75.
- Discuss with your healthcare provider if it's appropriate for you to continue getting screened if you're between the ages of 76 and 85. Consider your personal preferences, general health,

and previous screening experience while making your decision.

- Screening for colorectal cancer should no longer be done on anyone above 85.

If you choose to be screened with a test other than a colonoscopy, any abnormal test result needs to be followed up with a colonoscopy.

Screening guidelines for lung cancer
The American Cancer Society recommends yearly screening for lung cancer with a low-dose CT (LDCT) scan for people ages 50 to 80 who:

- Have at least 20 pack years of smoking history, or used to smoke.

- One pack, or around 20 cigarettes, smoked every day for a year is equivalent to one pack-year. For instance, smoking one pack per day for twenty years or two packs per day for ten years could result in a 20-pack-year history.

Before choosing to be screened, people should speak with a medical professional about the goals, procedures, limitations, and potential risks of screening as well as its benefits.

Counselling on quitting should be provided to smokers who are still in the habit, together with resources and initiatives to help them.

People should not be screened if they have serious health problems that will likely limit how long they will live, or if they won't be able to or won't want to get treatment if lung cancer is found.

Screening Guidelines for Skin Cancer

Routine screening for skin cancer

Experts do not recommend skin cancer screenings for most people. They don't recommend them if you have no history of skin cancer.

The U.S. Preventive Services Task Force (USPSTF) concluded that there is not enough evidence to recommend for or against routine screening total body examination by a doctor to find skin cancers early. Those without a history of skin cancer and any suspicious moles or other areas should follow this recommendation.

Checking your skin for moles regularly will help you find any suspicious changes. Be sure to check less visible areas of your skin like the soles of your feet. Tell your doctor about any unusual moles or changes in yours.

Signs and Symptoms to be Aware of

Different types of cancer can cause many different signs and symptoms. Sometimes, certain body parts, like our stomach or skin, are affected by the symptoms. However, general signs such as weight loss, fatigue, or unbearable pain may also occur.

A lump is one of the less well-known possible signs of cancer. They are not, however, more significant or likely to have cancer as a result of this. It is important to get any possible symptoms of cancer checked out.

People can be affected by cancer in different ways. Different people may experience different types of symptoms, and some people may not experience any symptoms at all. So, you don't need to remember all the signs and symptoms of cancer.

It's important to be aware of what is normal for you and speak to your doctor if you notice any unusual changes or something that won't go away. This can help to diagnose cancer at an early stage when treatment is more likely to be successful.

Chapter 3

Risk Factors: Identifying and Assessing Your Vulnerability

This chapter will look at the common risk factors associated with development, focusing on elements in the workplace and environment that may make a person vulnerable to the disease.

Discussion of common risk factors

The complex disease known as cancer may be influenced by a wide range of risk factors. To reduce your vulnerability to cancer, it's necessary to be aware of these risk factors and adopt ways to avoid them. The following are a few of the most common risk factors:

a. Age and Gender: Certain gender-specific traits, such as hormone imbalances and previous reproductive experiences, can increase your chance of developing cancer as you age.

Genetic Factors: The risk of ovarian, breast, and other cancers is markedly increased by certain inherited gene mutations, such as those affecting BRCA1 or BRCA2.

c. Lifestyle Choices: Long-term exposure to the sun without protection, poor diets deficient in fruits and vegetables, sedentary lifestyles with little exercise, and alcohol and tobacco use can all lead to the development of cancer.

d. Chronic Infections: Human papillomavirus (HPV), hepatitis B and C, and HIV are among the viruses that can lead to the increased risk of developing certain types of cancers.

Environmental and Occupational Factors

In addition to the standard risk factors already listed, exposure to environmental and occupational hazards can also result in the development of cancer. These factors, although preventable to some extent, can significantly increase a person's vulnerability. Now let's go into a few of these risk factors:

A. Air pollution

Air pollution, which is brought on by burning fossil fuels, car exhaust fumes, and industrial emissions, has been linked to a higher chance of developing lung, breast, and bladder cancers, among other medical conditions. Polluted air contains particulate matter and other hazardous substances that might enter the respiratory system and perhaps disrupt DNA, which could promote the growth of cancer cells.

B. Exposure to Harmful Chemicals

Certain chemicals used in agriculture, manufacturing, and domestic items might cause cancer. For instance, asbestos has been linked to mesothelioma and lung cancer and is frequently used in construction. Repetitive or high exposure to pesticides, solvents, heavy metals, and chemicals such as benzene found in petrol has been shown to increase the risk of cancer.

C. Radiation Exposure

Radiation from nuclear power plants, X-rays, and UV radiation from the sun or tanning salons are examples of ionising radiation that can greatly increase the chance of acquiring cancer. Long-term ionising radiation exposure can damage DNA and reduce a cell's ability to function properly, both of which can contribute to the development of cancer.

It is imperative to take the necessary safety precautions to minimise exposure to these environmental and occupational hazards wherever possible. You might lower your vulnerability to cancer caused by these risk factors by using protective equipment, strictly following safety guidelines and regulations, using technology responsibly, advocating for strict laws and cleaner air, and other measures.

Occupational hazards

Occupational hazards are risks and dangers that people may experience at work that raise their risk of developing cancer. It is essential to be aware of common carcinogens found in different professions and adopt protective measures to minimise exposure. By being aware of the particular hazards related to your line of work, you can prevent them from developing cancer.

Common Carcinogens in Different Professions

A. The Building Sector
 Asbestos: Asbestos is known to cause cancer and has been connected to lung cancer, mesothelioma, and other respiratory disorders. Workers engaged in building, demolition, and remodelling operations may be exposed to asbestos.

Silica: Breathing in silica dust increases the chance of getting silicosis and lung cancer in those who work in the construction, mining, or stone-cutting industries.

Benzene is a dangerous chemical that construction workers may come into contact with. It has been linked to cancer and leukaemia.

B. Radiation in the Healthcare Sector: During X-rays, CT scans, and other imaging procedures, medical professionals, including radiologists and radiologic technicians, are exposed to ionising radiation, which raises their chance of developing cancer.

Chemotherapy Drugs: Those who work with chemotherapy drugs in the medical field may come into contact with dangerous substances, which could increase their chance of developing certain cancers.

C. Agriculture and Farming
Pesticides: Agricultural workers and farmers may come into contact with pesticides, some

of which have been linked to cancer. A long period of exposure to specific medications may raise the chance of getting some cancers.

UV Radiation: Long-term exposure to UV light may increase the risk of skin cancer among farmers and other outdoor workers who spend a lot of time in the sun.

Protective Measures to Minimise Exposure

Reducing the number of chemicals in your surroundings that may be harmful is essential to lowering your risk of developing cancer. Chemicals included in many cosmetics, plastics, household cleaning goods, and pesticides can raise your risk of developing cancer. By following these safety measures, you can lower your risk.

Make sure you have the right protection at work if your job places you near possible carcinogens. Recognise the risks involved in your profession and adhere to safety regulations. Follow your employer's instructions and put on the proper safety equipment, such as goggles, a mask, or gloves. Maintain a secure and safe working environment by taking proactive steps to reduce risks.

The adoption of the suggested preventive measures can significantly reduce the chance of acquiring occupational cancer. People need to be well informed of the risks related to their line of work and proceed with extreme caution. These may consist of:

1. Use proper Protective Equipment PPE. Wearing appropriate gloves, masks, goggles, and other protective gear can prevent direct contact with hazardous materials, reducing the risk of exposure.

2. Adhering to the Safety Instructions. The dangers linked with carcinogenic

compounds at work can be reduced by following safety procedures and rules.

3. Implementing Proper Ventilation. At work, having the right ventilation systems installed can help get rid of dangerous chemicals, dust, and fumes, lowering the chance of exposure.

4. Regular Health Check-ups. Regular medical examinations and screenings can help detect any early signs of occupational diseases, allowing for prompt interventions and reducing the chances of cancer progression.

5. Advocating for Workplace Safety
By alerting their employers to any potential risks, workers should take the initiative to advocate for safe working conditions.

6. Education on Harmful Pollutants and Chemicals.

Stay informed about harmful pollutants and chemicals in your surroundings.

Be aware of the substances and chemicals that are present in your environment. Research to know more about the possible risks connected to particular goods or medications. Read product labels carefully, and if at all possible, select non-toxic, environmentally friendly items. Consider using natural cleaning products, organic cosmetics, and pesticide-free home gardening techniques.

Those who take preventive steps and are aware of common carcinogens in various industries can greatly lower their risk of developing occupational cancers. Companies and employees must prioritise occupational safety and well-being to create a cancer-free and healthy work environment.

Tobacco and Alcohol

A. Risks of Smoking and Tobacco Use

Smoking and tobacco use are among the leading causes of various types of cancer, including lung, throat, mouth, pancreas, bladder, and kidney cancer. The risk of cancer is greatly increased by tobacco smoke since it contains toxic ingredients like tar, nicotine, and other carcinogens. Smoking not only causes lung illnesses and cancer but also heart problems and other major health issues. Knowing the dangers of smoking and using tobacco is crucial if you want to be aware of the grave implications these habits may have on your health.

B. Recommended Limits for Alcohol Consumption

Drinking alcohol does not carry many serious dangers as long as it is consumed within recommended limits. However, excessive and persistent drinking can raise the risk of some cancers, including those of the mouth, throat, liver, breast, and lung cancer. It is essential to adhere to the following advice:

For men: it is advised that men limit their alcohol intake to two standard drinks per day.

For women: it is recommended to consume no more than one standard drink per day.

You can dramatically lower your risk of alcohol-related cancers and other related health issues by adhering to these guidelines.

Strategies for Quitting Smoking or Reducing Alcohol Intake

Quitting Smoking

Giving up smoking is one of the best things you can do to lower your risk of cancer. Some strategies to help you stop smoking are as follows:

Establish a quit date and stick to it. Set a date to quit smoking and demonstrate to yourself that you are committed to living a healthier lifestyle.

Seek assistance from others. Tell your close friends, family, and medical professionals that you have decided to give up smoking. Seek their assistance; they could provide you with motivation, guidance, and encouragement along the process.

Use nicotine replacement therapy or NRT. NRT, such as nicotine patches or gum, may reduce cravings and the symptoms of withdrawal associated with quitting smoking. Consult your physician to determine which kind of NRT is right for you.

Consider joining a smoking cessation program or support group. Consider registering for a programme or support group aimed at quitting smoking. These programmes offer psychological therapy, professional counselling, and effective smoking cessation strategies.

B. Reducing alcohol intake

If you are concerned about your alcohol consumption and its potential impact on your health, here are some strategies to help you reduce your alcohol intake:

Set clear goals. You can determine your desired reduction in alcohol consumption and set specific, achievable goals along the way.

Identify your triggers. Recognise what situations, emotions, or environments lead you to this negative habit. As you identify these triggers, you can develop alternative coping mechanisms and healthier habits.

Consult a professional. If you're struggling to quit your drinking habits, you can receive personal assistance and guidance from medical professionals or addiction therapists.

Engage in alternative activities. You can replace drinking with enjoyable, stress-relieving, and profitable hobbies. Fun activities, hobbies, and spending time with loved ones are all good strategies to divert your attention from drinking alcohol.

One of the most important steps in preventing cancer is realising the risks associated with alcohol and tobacco use. You can significantly lower your chance of developing cancer by adhering to recommended alcohol consumption guidelines and using possible approaches to quit smoking or reduce your drinking habits. You have the power to make positive changes that will benefit your health and ultimately contribute to a cancer-free life.

Chapter 4

Genetic Factors and Hereditary Cancer Syndromes

In this chapter, common hereditary cancer syndromes will be discussed, along with the role that genetic factors play in the development of cancer. With a greater understanding of these inherited factors, people and their families can realise their risks and take the necessary precautions.

Recognising the role of genetics in the development of cancer

Environmental and genetic factors have a role in the complex disease known as cancer. Even while food, radiation exposure, and tobacco use are key environmental influences, genetic factors also play a role in the development of cancer. A person's vulnerability to specific types of cancer can be increased by specific gene abnormalities, which are referred to as genetic factors. These mutations can be inherited or acquired by a person over their lifetime.

Cancer is a hereditary disease. Changes in genes that regulate cell division and growth are the root cause of it. Your body's cells are its fundamental units. Your genes function as an instruction manual and are replicated in every cell.

DNA segments called genes are responsible for carrying instructions needed to produce one or more proteins. Numerous genetic and DNA modifications—also referred to as variations, mutations, or alterations—have been discovered by scientists to contribute to the initiation, growth, and spread of cancer.

Because random errors in our DNA occur when our cells grow, cancer-related changes in genetics may arise. Carcinogens in our surroundings, such as human papillomavirus (HPV), chemicals in tobacco smoke, and UV rays from the sun, change our DNA; these genes were passed down from one of our parents.

DNA changes, whether caused by a random mistake or by a carcinogen, can happen throughout our lives and even in the womb. The majority of genetic changes don't cause harm on their own, but over many years, a buildup of these changes can cause healthy cells to become dangerous. The vast majority of cancers occur by chance as a result of this process over time.

Common hereditary cancer syndromes

Cancer itself cannot be passed down from parents to children. Moreover, genetic tumour cells are not transmissible. However, if a genetic change that raises the risk of cancer is found in a parent's sperm or egg, it can be inherited.

A child's risk of developing breast cancer and multiple other types of cancer is significantly increased if their parent carries a mutant copy of the BRCA1 or BRCA2 gene.

A family member with a higher-than-average risk of developing a particular type of cancer is said to have familial cancer syndrome, also known as hereditary cancer syndrome. Genes linked to cancer that have inherited genetic variations are the source of family cancer syndromes. Some family cancer syndromes cause people to either have various non-cancer health concerns or develop cancer at a young age.

For this reason, cancer may seem to run in families at times. Genetic changes inherited from parents may be the cause of up to 10% of cancer cases. It is not a guarantee that you will develop cancer if you inherit a change in genetics linked to cancer. It indicates a higher chance of developing cancer.

Not every cancer that seems to "run in families" has a family cancer syndrome as its cause. The same type of cancer may develop in family members due to common habits or environments, such as tobacco smoking or exposure to air pollution.

Also, family members may develop common cancers, such as prostate cancer, just by chance. Cancer can also run in a family if family members have a combination of many genetic variants that each have a very small cancer risk.

Chapter 5

Protective Measures: Practical Steps to Minimise Cancer Risks

Our battle against cancer depends heavily on taking precautions that lower our exposure to possible threats. The key to reducing the risk of cancer is regular physical activity and exercise. You'll find steps in this chapter that you can take every day to protect yourself and reduce your risk of cancer. You will be taking a significant stride towards safeguarding your well-being by embracing these protective measures. We'll discuss the importance of maintaining a healthy weight and how obesity increases the chance of getting cancer. We'll also provide you with helpful tips on how to control your weight to avoid developing cancer.

Promoting a Healthy Lifestyle (Healthy Diet and Nutrition)

A. Importance of a Balanced Diet

To protect yourself against cancer, you must maintain a balanced diet. A balanced diet contains every essential component—including vitamins, minerals, and elements—that our bodies need to operate at good efficiency. A well-rounded diet ensures that our immune system remains strong and capable of fighting off cancer cells. Maintaining a healthy weight also helps reduce the risk of other cancers, including breast, colorectal, and kidney cancer.

B. Foods to Include

We can significantly lower our risk of developing cancer by incorporating certain foods into our normal diet. Our nutrition plan should include the following essential meals:

1. Fruits and Vegetables: These should comprise a large portion of our meals every day. In addition to essential nutrients, eating a variety of colourful fruits and vegetables provides us with antioxidants, which protect our cells from damage.

2. Whole Grains: Consuming whole grains, such as quinoa, brown rice, and whole wheat bread, as opposed to processed grains, may help prevent cancer. Whole grains are rich in fibre, vitamins, and minerals that aid digestion and help maintain a healthy body.

3. Legumes: Legumes such as beans, lentils, and chickpeas are an excellent source of plant-based protein, fibre, and other essential elements. Consuming them in our diet can lower the risk of colorectal cancer as well as other cancers.

4. Lean Protein: Opt for lean sources of protein like skinless poultry, fish, and tofu, which provide the necessary amino acids for the body without adding excess fat. Your risk of developing cancer can also be reduced through consuming less red and processed meat.

C. Foods to Avoid

Eating a balanced diet is important, but so is limiting or avoiding certain foods to lower the risk of cancer. You should stay away from the following foods:

1. Processed Meats: Highly processed meats, such as sausages, bacon, and deli meats,

include chemicals like nitrates and nitrites that can increase the risk of colorectal cancer. Minimising their consumption is advisable.

2. Sugary Foods and Drinks: Eating and drinking a lot of sugar raises the risk of weight gain and obesity-related cancers, such as breast, liver, and pancreatic cancer. Limit your intake of sugar-filled foods and opt for healthier ones.

3. Unhealthy Fats: Cancer may develop as a result of trans fats, which are included in processed and fried foods, as well as saturated fats, which are found in fatty meats and full-fat dairy products. Replacing these with healthier fats like olive oil, avocados, and nuts is recommended.

4. Excessive Alcohol Consumption: Cutting back on alcohol is essential to preventing cancer. Among other cancers, alcohol consumption has been directly linked to an

increased risk of developing colon, breast, and liver cancers. The best course of action is to either cut back on alcohol consumption or abstain entirely.

D. Maintaining a Healthy Weight

Maintaining a healthy weight is crucial for overall health and well-being. Obesity not only negatively impacts our self-esteem and quality of life but also increases the risk of various types of cancer. It is important to strive for a healthy body mass index (BMI) through regular exercise and adopting a balanced, nutritious diet.

The Risk of Obesity in Cancer
It's commonly known that obesity increases the risk of several cancers, including endometrial, pancreatic, renal, breast, and colon cancers. Insomnia can lead to chronic inflammation, hormone imbalances, and insulin resistance, all of which contribute to the development of cancer cells.

Hormone imbalances in women can result from obesity, particularly from oestrogen, which has been linked to endometrial and breast cancers. Moreover, insulin resistance brought on by being overweight can raise blood levels of insulin and growth factors that resemble insulin, thus promoting the proliferation of cancer cells.

Men who are obese may have an increased risk of colorectal and prostate cancers. According to a study, having too much fat around the waist may contribute to the development of some cancers.

Tips for Weight Management

1. Incorporate Regular Exercise: Perform moderate-to-intense aerobic exercise for at least 150 minutes per week, or 75 minutes of such activity. Include strength training exercises twice a week to build muscle mass and boost metabolism.

2. Follow a Well-Balanced Diet: Ensure that you consume adequate amounts of fruits, vegetables, whole grains, lean meats, and healthy fats. Processed foods high in trans and saturated fats increase the risk of cancer and make you gain weight, so avoid them.

3. Get Adequate Sleep: Try to get seven to eight hours of good sleep every night. Inadequate sleep can cause hormone imbalances, increase appetites for unhealthy foods, and result in weight gain.

4. Limit Alcohol and Sugary Drinks: High consumption of sugary drinks and alcohol is linked to weight gain and an increased risk of certain cancers. Opt for water, herbal tea, or unsweetened beverages instead.

5. Be Mindful of Emotional Eating: Avoid using food as an escape from boredom, anxiety, or other emotions. Look for alternatives, such as exercising, practising

mindfulness, or asking friends and family for help.

6. Seek Professional Assistance: If controlling your weight proves to be difficult for you, think about consulting a certified dietician or other healthcare professional, or enrolling in a weight-management programme.

Keeping your weight within a healthy range can help you to proactively lower your risk of developing cancer by heeding these helpful guidelines. Small changes can make a big difference in protecting yourself against cancer. Remain committed to living a healthy lifestyle and value your well-being.

Chapter 6

Prevention Strategies for Specific Cancers

Although certain lifestyle choices may reduce your overall risk of cancer, it's important to remember that there is no guaranteed "cancer diet," exercise programme, "cancer-fighting superfood," or other silver bullet that may prevent cancer completely. Despite doing the right thing (i.e. maintaining an ideal weight, making healthy choices, etc.), men and women still tragically receive a breast cancer diagnosis due to circumstances beyond their control.

However, there are things listed below that you may do to potentially lower your risk of developing cancer and other dangerous diseases like diabetes and heart disease.

We've compiled tips and modifications supported by evidence to help lower your chance of developing cancer and other diseases.

Breast Cancer

Throughout a lifetime, numerous factors will influence your risk of breast cancer. While there are certain factors beyond your control, such as age or family history, you can reduce your risk of breast cancer by implementing the following preventive measures:

- Maintain a healthy weight.
- Engage in physical activity.

- Choose to either abstain from alcohol entirely or to use it moderately.
- If you are taking, or have been told to take, hormone replacement therapy or oral contraceptives (birth control pills), ask your doctor about the risks and find out if it is right for you.
- If at all possible, breastfeed your children.
- If you have a family history of breast cancer or inherited changes in your BRCA1 and BRCA2 genes, talk to your doctor about other ways to lower your risk.

Find Out Your Family History. Women who have a high risk of cancer in their families may need to take additional measures to reduce or control it. If your mother, sister, or other close relatives (including men) have had breast, ovarian, or prostate cancer, especially at a young age, you may be at an increased risk of developing breast cancer. A doctor or genetic counsellor can help you understand your family history of the disease.

Staying healthy throughout your life will lower your risk of developing cancer, and improve your chances of surviving cancer if it occurs.

Lung Cancer

It's not possible to avoid lung cancer. However, there are certain things you may do to potentially reduce your risk, like observing the risk factors under your control.

Stay away from tobacco

Avoiding secondhand smoke and quitting smoking are the best ways to lower your risk of developing lung cancer. Your damaged lung tissue will begin to heal itself if you quit smoking before a cancerous tumour appears. No matter what your age or how long you've smoked, quitting may lower your risk of lung cancer and help you live longer.

Avoid radon exposure
Lung cancer is largely caused by radon. If your home has to be tested and treated for radon, you can lower your exposure to the gas. For additional details,

Avoid or limit exposure to cancer-causing agents
Aside from the job, avoiding exposure to recognised carcinogens may also be beneficial. Workplace exposures to these kinds of hazards ought to be minimised for employees.

Eat a healthy diet
Lung cancer risk may also be lowered by eating a balanced diet high in fruits and vegetables. According to some research, a diet rich in fruits and vegetables may help prevent lung cancer in both smokers and non-smokers. However, the reduced risk of lung cancer caused by smoking would be

greater than any benefit that fruits and vegetables may have.

Colorectal Cancer

Age, race, uncommon inherited genetic diseases, family history, and personal history are among the many risk factors for colon cancer that may be changed, but many others cannot. These are the most effective strategies for preventing colon cancer.

Get Screened

The most effective strategy to protect against colon cancer is to have screening tests regularly. By identifying abnormal growths called polyps that have the potential to develop into cancer, it can detect the disease early on, when it is most curable.

Maintain a Healthy Weight

Being overweight is the only factor that increases one's overall risk of cancer, other than smoking. Obesity and weight growth have been linked to at least 13 different cancers, including colon cancer. Attempting to stop gaining weight is an excellent first step if you've gained weight, as it has its health benefits.

Don't Smoke
Quitting smoking is the best thing you can do for your health—it barely needs to be said. Colon cancer is among the fifteen cancers that are caused by smoking. In addition, it raises the risk of developing emphysema, heart disease, and stroke, among other dangerous illnesses.

Be Physically Active
It's hard to beat regular activity. It improves mental health and reduces the chance of some major illnesses, such as colon cancer. While any exercise is better than none at all, it's a good idea to aim for at least 30 minutes a day of moderate exercise. Pick activities you enjoy doing, such as

gardening, dancing, cycling, or brisk walking.

Limit alcohol – Zero is best
The risk of breast and colon cancers can increase with alcohol consumption, even in small amounts. Furthermore, abstaining from alcohol is generally the healthiest option given its additional hazards.

Limit Red Meat, especially Processed Meat
Eating a lot of red meat, such as pig, steak, and hamburgers, raises the risk of colon cancer. Furthermore, processed meats like bologna, sausage and bacon increase risk even further. Aim to eat no more than three servings each week. Less is even preferable.

Vitamins, calcium, and magnesium
According to some studies, vitamin D, which can be obtained from sun exposure, specific food, or vitamin supplements, may reduce the risk of colorectal cancer. Low vitamin D levels have been linked in studies to a higher

risk of colorectal cancer and other cancers. Most doctors do not now advise this as a way to lower the risk of colorectal cancer because of concerns that excessive sun exposure can cause skin cancer. If taking a supplement higher in vitamin D can help prevent colorectal cancer, more research is required to make that decision.

Prostate Cancer
Although there is no one way to prevent prostate cancer, many people might wonder how to do so. Treating health problems that already exist or maintaining good health as you age can reduce your risk. Prostate cancer does, however, have some inevitable risk factors, just like any other cancer.

Things You Cannot Change: genes, Age, and Race
Essentially, prostate cancer is a "disease of ageing." The likelihood of having prostate cancer rises with age. Genetics and race are important factors as well. If you are African

American, your chances of developing prostate cancer are double those of white American men. You are more likely to develop prostate cancer if your father, brother, or several other blood relatives did.

If you have these risk factors, it may be difficult to prevent prostate cancer, but regular screenings can help make sure that if cancer does develop, it is identified and treated as soon as possible.

Things You Can Change:
Improve your diet (eat more fruits and vegetables and reduce fat intake)
Stay sexually active
Stop smoking and drink less
Maintain a healthy weight
Increase your Vitamin D
Get regular exercise

Skin Cancer

The best way to prevent skin cancer is to protect your skin from the sun and protect yourself against harmful UV radiation.

To protect yourself from skin cancer:

Stay out of the sun as much as possible between 10 a.m. and 4 p.m.
Avoid tanning, and never use UV tanning beds.
Cover up with long sleeves, long pants or a long skirt, a hat, and sunglasses
Perform regular skin self-exams to detect skin cancer early, when it's most treatable, and see a board-certified dermatologist if you notice new or suspicious spots on your skin,
Use sunscreen with SPF 15 or higher
Don't get sunburned.
Don't use indoor tanning machines
Check your skin for changes regularly

Other Common Cancers

In addition to colorectal, prostate, breast, lung, and skin cancers, many additional cancer types also need to be addressed to lower the rate of cancer. For instance, routine cervical cancer screenings, particularly Pap tests, can help in the prevention of cancer. It is also advised that men and women get the human papillomavirus (HPV) vaccine to guard against HPV strains that have been linked to cancer. Reducing the risk factors for chronic hepatitis B and hepatitis C infections, such as sharing needles, unsafe injection practices, and unprotected sex, can help prevent liver cancer.

Chapter 7

The Future of Cancer Prevention and Research

Cancer research and breakthroughs hold immense significance in the quest for a cancer-free world. These scientific endeavours not only deepen our understanding of cancer development and progression but also pave the way for innovative treatments and prevention strategies. Research is essential to the development of targeted therapies, survivability rates, and early detection. It serves as the cornerstone for further advancements, instilling optimism and hope in cancer patients and their loved ones

However, the most effective primary prevention of cancer that works best is based on whole-of-government strategies that include actions to modify personal community behaviour together with laws, regulations, and fiscal policies. Evidence on particular risk factors should be included in public health advocacy and health promotion initiatives.

Ways People Can Contribute to Cancer Research and Advocacy

Even though scientists and medical professionals are crucial to the cause, people like you may help drive cancer research forward. Here are a few key ways you can contribute:

Participate in Clinical Trials: Clinical trials are the backbone of cancer research, offering the chance to test new treatments and potential remedies. As you volunteer for these trials, you not only contribute to the advancement of science but also provide crucial insights that may benefit future patients.

Support Fundraising Initiatives: Many cancer research institutions depend on donations and public support to fund their endeavours. To raise funds for cancer research, you can organise your events, take part in fundraisers, or donate to reputable charities. Every contribution makes a difference, no matter how small.

Raise Awareness and Education: Share information about cancer prevention, the importance of early detection, and available services with your friends, family, and community. Encourage them to participate in cancer research initiatives, adopt healthier lifestyles, and get frequent checkups. Education is a powerful tool in the fight against cancer.

Inspiring Readers to Become Advocates in Their Communities

Taking up the role of an advocate is a powerful method to fight cancer in your community. You can make a tangible change. Encourage others to follow suit by acting and thinking through the next steps.

Join Local Cancer Organizations: Find local cancer organisations or support groups that align with your interests. One way to support local advocacy initiatives is to actively participate in their events and programmes, offer support to cancer patients, and help raise awareness in your community.

Use Social Media Platforms: Utilise social media to its fullest potential to spread your message and increase awareness of critical cancer-related topics. Educate people by sharing stories, words of encouragement, and educational materials to encourage them to prevent cancer and to support ongoing research.

Engage with Policy Makers: Discuss issues relating to cancer with your government officials, take part in open forums, and express your concerns. Promote the adoption of policies that prioritise cancer prevention, increase funding for research, and improve access to healthcare. Your involvement has the potential to impact positive change on a bigger scale.

The combined efforts of people, organisations, and communities will shape future directions in cancer prevention and research. We can create a future where cancer is preventable and treatable by recognizing the importance of ongoing research and breakthroughs, contributing actively to cancer research and advocacy, and inspiring others to join the cause. Let us unite in our quest for a cancer-free world, one that offers hope, compassion, and support to all those affected by this deadly disease. Together, we can make a difference. When we work together, we can make a difference.

Cancer research is crucial to the goal of eliminating the disease worldwide. These research projects not only improve our understanding of the causes and progression of cancer but also make it easier to create new treatments and precautionary measures. Research is essential to the development of customised treatments, survivability rates, and early diagnosis techniques. It serves as the cornerstone for further advancements, instilling optimism and hope in cancer patients and their loved ones.

Ways People Can Contribute to Cancer Research and Advocacy

Even though scientists and medical professionals are crucial to the cause, people like you may help progress cancer research. Here are a few key ways you can contribute:

Participate in Clinical Trials: Clinical trials are the mainstay of cancer research, offering the chance to test new treatments and potential remedies. In addition to improving science, taking part in these trials provides vital information that may benefit patients in the future.

Support Fundraising Initiatives: Many cancer research institutions depend on donations and public support to fund their operations. To raise funds for cancer research, you can organise your events, take part in fundraisers, or donate to reputable charities. Every contribution matters, no matter how small.

Raise Awareness and Education: Share information about cancer prevention, the importance of early detection, and available services with your friends, family, and community. Encourage people to participate in cancer research initiatives, adopt healthier lifestyles, and get frequent checkups. Education is a powerful tool in the fight against cancer.

Inspiring Readers to Become Advocates in Their Communities

Taking up the role of an advocate is a powerful method to fight cancer in your neighbourhood. You can effect real change. Consider the following steps by inspiring others and taking action.

Join Local Cancer Organizations: Find groups or local cancer organisations that match your interests. One way to support local advocacy initiatives is to actively participate in their events and programmes, offer support to cancer patients, and help raise awareness in your community.

Utilise Social Media Platforms: Utilise social media to its fullest potential to spread your message and increase awareness of critical cancer-related topics. Educate people by sharing stories, words of encouragement, and educational materials to encourage them to take proactive steps towards cancer prevention and to support ongoing research.

Engage with Policy Makers: Discuss issues relating to cancer with your government officials, take part in open forums, and express your concerns. Promote the adoption of policies that prioritise cancer prevention, increase funding for research, and improve access to healthcare. Your involvement has the potential to impact positive change on a bigger scale.

The future of cancer prevention and research is reliant on the collective efforts of people, communities, and organisations. Through our active participation in cancer advocacy, understanding of the significance of ongoing research and advancements, and motivating others to support the cause, we can build a future in which cancer is treated and prevented. Let us unite in our quest for a cancer-free world, one that offers hope, compassion, and support to all those affected by this deadly disease. Together, we can make a difference.

Chapter 8

Hope for a Cancer-free Future

Positive trends for certain cancers (e.g. lung cancer) will be a reflection of the progress made in tobacco control. Further efforts to reduce cancer mortality may be possible in the future if efforts are made to control alcohol consumption, infections, and associated neoplasms, as well as to enhance screening, early detection, and treatment outcomes. The chance of developing cancer can be considerably reduced by consistently following these preventative measures.

However, even with our best efforts, cancer can sometimes strike unexpectedly. It is essential to remember that no person should shoulder the burden of a cancer diagnosis alone. Medical advancements have revolutionised cancer treatment, and remarkable progress has been made in recent years. For people afflicted with this disease, there is now greater hope than ever before.

From ground-breaking immunotherapies to targeted therapies and precision medicine, cancer treatments are becoming more personalised and effective. Experts are relentlessly striving to understand cancer at its core, unravelling the fundamental causes of cancer, reassembling its complex systems, and developing new methods for treating it. Positive results have raised hopes for better outcomes for cancer patients.

Additionally, early detection and awareness are also necessary to raise survival rates.

Regular screening and checkups can help identify cancer at its early stage when it is still treatable. Communities are coming together, raising awareness and funds for research, making sure everyone has access to quality cancer care and support.

As we look to the future, we must continue to advocate for research funding, support those affected by cancer, and shatter the stigma surrounding the disease. We can empower people, families, and communities to take control of their health by doing this and making prevention and early detection a top priority.

I hope that after reading this, you will remain well-informed, careful, and optimistic. We are not fighting cancer alone, and if we work together, we can work towards a cancer-free future. Let us hold onto hope, for it is hope that drives us to take action, sparks new ideas, and ultimately, brings us closer to a world without cancer.

Last but not least, I would like to thank you for taking the time to read this book. Hopefully, the facts and thoughts shared on these pages have assisted you in making wise decisions regarding cancer prevention. Remember always that information truly is power and that everything is possible when you have it.

Let's hope for a brighter tomorrow where cancer will be but a distant memory and every one of us may enjoy life to the fullest without having to worry about this dreadful disease. May hope always illuminate your path, and may you walk carefully and safely.

Sources:
American Cancer Society: "Breast Cancer Symptoms: What You Need to

Know," "Learn about Cancer: Breast Cancer."

National Cancer Institute: "Breast Cancer."

Canadian Cancer Society: "Symptoms of breast cancer."

National Cancer Institute Center for Cancer Research: "Angiosarcoma."

Skin Cancer Foundation. Skin & Skin News. Ask the Expert: Is There a Skin Cancer Crisis in People of Color? (https://www.skincancer.org/blog/ask-the-expert-is-there-a-skin-cancer-crisis-in-people-of-color/) Accessed 10/21/2023.

American Academy of Dermatology. Skin Cancer. (https://www.aad.org/media/stats-skin-cancer)
Accessed 10/21/2023.

National Cancer Institute: The Surveillance, Epidemiology, and End Results (SEER) Program. Cancer Stat Facts: Lung and Bronchus Cancer (https://seer.cancer.gov/statfacts/html/lungb.html). Accessed 10/28/2022.

Centres for Disease Control and Prevention. Multiple pages were reviewed for this article (https://www.cdc.gov/cancer/colorectal/basic_info/). Accessed 10/28/2022.

NCCN guidelines for patients: Colon cancer. National Comprehensive Cancer Network. https://www.NCCN.org/patients. Accessed Nov. 14, 2023.

Prostate cancer. National Comprehensive Cancer Network. https://www.nccn.org/professionals/physician_gls/default.aspx. Accessed Nov. 19, 2023.

Your Disease Risk

Zuum Health Tracker

Www.bcrf.org

8ight Ways to Prevent Cancer
SmokeFree.gov

NIH Body Mass Index Calculator

National Cancer Institute

American Cancer Society

CDC–Family Health History

www.ingramcontent.com/pod-product-compliance
Lightning Source LLC
Chambersburg PA
CBHW070911260726

48661CB00004B/1699